THE
MATERIA M
OF
SOME MORE
IMPORTANT REMEDIES

H.C. Allen, M.D.

B. JAIN PUBLISHERS (P) LTD.
An ISO 9001 : 2000 Certified Company
USA—Europe—India

THE MATERIA MEDICA OF SOME MORE IMPORTANT REMEDIES

Revised Edition: 2000
Reprint Edition: 2008

Published by Kuldeep Jain for
B. JAIN PUBLISHERS (P) LTD.
An ISO 9001 : 2000 Certified Company
1921/10, Chuna Mandi, Paharganj, New Delhi 110 055 (INDIA)
Tel.: 91-11-2358 0800, 2358 1100, 2358 1300, 2358 3100
Fax: 91-11-2358 0471 • Email: info@bjain.com
Website: www.bjainbooks.com

Printed in India by
Akash Press

ISBN: 978-81-319-0594-6

CONTENTS

CONTENTS

ADRENALIN (Sarcode)

Extr. of Suprarenal bodies $C_3H_3A_2O_1$

Mental Generals

- Despondent and nervous; lack of interest in anything; no ambition; disinclination for mental work; absence of "grit."
- Aversion to mental work, cannot concentrate thoughts.

Head

- Hot headache in left side, extending to right, < by reading and in morning, with a feeling as though the eyes were strained.
- Frontal headache, supraorbital, with congested nose and eyes.
- Burning heat in head, feeling as though he wanted to open eyes wide.
- Headache extending all over head but < on left side and over eyes across forehead.
- Severe pain > by pressure on the eyes.
- Headache extending to the ears. All headaches are < in. the afternoon or evening; in the evening they appear about 7 P.M. and last until relieved by walk in the open air or sleep.

- If headache appears in the afternoon the time is 3 P.M., always > by walk in the open air, and some-what relieved by eating and sleeping, but not so completely as by walk in the open air.
- Neuralgic headache; pains start from base of brain, go forward over the head to front and sides; pains are first shooting and seem to be just under the scalp, appear at 11 A.M. and last until 3 or 4 P.M. and disappear by eating, in open air, < in close, warm room.
- Dull aching in the eyeballs with headache, > by pressure and by rubbing the eyes.
- Headache coming on at 11 A.M., lasting until 12-30 at night, > by eating.
- Dull feeling in the head from 3 to 6 P.M.

Eyes

- Strained feeling, congested, feeling as though he wanted to open them wide or press upon them.
- Pain in the right eye. Pressure on the eyes and opening them wide > the headache.
- Aching in eyeballs, > by pressure and rubbing.

Ears

- Aching in the left ear accompanies the headache; sharp pain in both ears at times.

  Itching and tickling in right ear, > by boring into ear with finger.

Nose

- On going out into the cold air has a copious watery nasal discharge, < on right side; when indoors, the nose feels full and stopped up.
- Slight stuffiness in the nose, with full feeling at the root of the nose.

Face

- Feels flushed but is not red.
- Flushes of heat over face and head; flushed throughout evening.

Mouth

- Bad taste on waking.
- Tongue coated white, red edge and tip.

Throat

- Vocal cords inflamed; laryngeal catarrh, profuse secretion from the pharyngeal glands of whitish gelatinous mucus which was difficult to loosen.

Respiratory System

- Cough, from irritation in suprasternal fossa.
- Increase of respiratory movements, soon followed by suffocation and death from paralysis of medulla and pneumogastric (crude drugs).

Gastro-intestinal System

- Appetite increased.
- Sensation of nausea as though he would vomit.
- Nausea before meals, though appetite is good when he once began to eat.
- Appetite increased; ravenous hunger.
- Stool loose, brown, semi-solid, passed quickly, with foetid odour.
- Sudden spluttering diarrhoea; all over in a minute, followed with burning in anus.

Urinary System

- Strong odour, hot and scalding; frequent, profuse, pale.
- Burning before and during micturition.

- Crystals of sodium oxalate increased while sodium urate appeared during the proving, and was very prominent, no casts.
- Haematuria with severe pain in the renal region; cured.
- Urine more frequent than usual.
- Sexual desire increased, without erections.
- Erections; lascivious dreams all night causing waking from sleep.
- Emissions in early morning without any bad effects.

Back

- Pain especially on the left side; better by sitting up straight or lying straight.

Extremities

- Slight rheumatic pains coming and going down leg.
- Arms and legs go to sleep easily; numbness and tingling from below upwards.
- Corns on the toes.
- Rheumatic pains in left elbow and little finger on waking.
- Legs tired and ache, especially in the calves and below the knees.
- Ankles feel weak and tired.
- Painful swelling on first finger of right hand, resulting in a felon.
- Tired aching in arms and legs on walking.

Tissues

- Prolonged contraction of the general muscular system. Repeated injections cause atheroma and heart lesions in animals.
- The skin becomes bronzed; great loss of strength; rapid

emaciation; exceedingly rapid pulse; irregular intermiting heart beats; general marked anaemia.

Sleep

- Great sleepiness and drowsiness.
- Dulness and sleepiness from 3 to 6 P.M.

BACILLINUM

A Maceration of a Typical Tuberculous Lung

Mental Generals

- Taciturn, sulky, snappish, fretty, irritable, morose, depressed and melancholic even to insanity.
- Fretful ailing, whines and complains; mind given to be frightened particularly by dogs.

Head

- Severe headache, deep in, recurring from time to time, compelling quiet fixedness; < shaking head.
- Terrible pain in head as if he had a tight hoop of iron around it; trembling of hands; sensation of damp clothes on spine; absolute sleeplessness.
- Alopecia areata.

Eyes

- Eczematous condition of eyelids.

Face

- Indolent, angry pimples on 1. cheek, breaking out from time to time and persisting for many weeks.

Teeth

- Grinds teeth in sleep.
- Imperfectly developed teeth.

Respiratory System

- Hard cough, shaking patient, more during sleep, but it did not waken him.
- Single cough on rising from bed in morning.
- Cough waking him in night; easy expectoration.
- Sharp pain in precordial region arresting breathing.
- Very sharp pain in left scapula, < lying down in bed at night, > by warmth.

Gastro-intestinal System

- Windy dyspepsia, with pinching pains under ribs of r.side in mammary line.
- Fever, emaciation, abdominal pains and discomfort, restless at night, glands of both groins enlarged and indurated; cries out in sleep; strawberry tongue.
- Tabes mesenterica; talks in sleep; grinds teeth; appetite poor; hands blue : indurated and palpable glands everywhere; drum belly; spleen region bulging out.
- Inguinal glands indurated and visible; excessive sweats; chronic diarrhoea.
- Obstinate constipation.
- Passes much ill-smelling flatus.
- Stitch-like pain through piles.

Urinary System

- Increased quantity of urine, pale, with white sediment.
- Has to rise several times in night to urinate.

Glands

- Glands of neck enlarged and tender.

Lower Limbs

- Tubercular inflammation of knee.

Generalities

- Great weakness, did not want to be disturbed.

Sleep

- Drowsy during day; restless at night; many dreams.

Fever

- Flush of heat (soon after the dose), some perspiration, severe headache deep in.

CHOLESTERINUM

Cholesterine $C_{26}H_{44}O$

Swan appears to have taken his hint from burnett's work and potentized the remedy, using a gall-stone for his preparations. Like many of the rest of the nosodes originally introduced by Swan, the work was necessarily empirical, yet he affirms after much experience that it is "almost a specific for gall-stone colic; relieves the distress at once." And this after failure with Nux-v., Cinchona, Carduus, Podophyllum and other apparently well-selected remedies.

Yingling reports some cures of gall-stone colic and other diseases of the liver in the *Medical Advance,* page 549, August, 1908.

Clarke says, it is found in the blood, in the brain, the yolk of eggs, seeds and buds of plants, but is most abundant in the bile and biliary calculi. It occurs in the form of crystals with a mother-of pearl lustre, and is fatty to the touch. It is soluble in both alcohol and ether.

Ameke claimed to have derived great advantage from its use in cases diagnosed as cancer of the liver, or in such obstinate engorgements that malignancy was suspected.

Burnett claims to have twice cured cancer of the liver with it, and "in hepatic engorgements that by reason of their intractable and slow yielding to well-selected remedies make one think interrogationally of cancer." In such conditions, where the diagnosis is in doubt, especially if the patient has been subjected to repeated attacks of biliary colic, Cholesterinum, he claims, is very satisfactory and at times its action even striking.

Yingling reports the following cases :

1st case

Attacks come suddenly and cease suddenly.

Pain is pushing in region of gall duct.

Marked acidity of stomach since last attack.

No appetite; food nauseates.

Regions of liver sore, sensitive to touch or jar, <lying on the sides.

2nd case

Vomits bile and becomes very yellow.

Liver very sensitive and sore : pressure in front or behind very painful, worse in region of gall duct.

Bending or any sudden motion aggravates.

Cholesterinum 2m. not only promptly relieved acute attacks, but has effected a practical cure."'

ELECTRICTAS
(Atmospheric and Static)

Caspari and his colleagues obtained the symptoms caused by Electrcity, natural and artificial, and was first published in **hom. Bibliot.** Later it appears in Jahr and has recently been republished, with additions by Clarks. Every medical man knows the extreme susceptibility of some persons to the electric fluid and the sufferings they experience on the approach of, and during, a thunder-storm, or the contact of an electric current.

The potencies are prepared from milk sugar which has been saturated with the current.

Characteristics - Intense nervous anxiety; timid, fearful, sighing : screams through nervous fear; paroxysms of weeping.

Dreads the approach of a thunder-storm; suffers mental torture before and during an electric storm.

Heaviness and paralysis of limbs and entire body, feels as if she weighted a ton.

Electricity should not be used nor electro-thermal baths taken when suffering from a cold, especially if the chest be involved; fatal results have followed.

Relations - Antidote : Morphia acetate, especially the potency. Clarke says : "I have found Phosphorus the best antidote to the effects of storms."

Compare - The X-ray, Psor., Tub. to remove the susceptibility.

ELECTRICITY

Mental Generals

- Weeping, timid, fearful; sighing; crying out through nervous fear.
- Paroxysms of oppressive anxiety.
- Dread at the approach of a thunder-storm; fear; internal anguish, especially of chest; nervous agitation.

- Involuntary hysterical laughter. Rage. Ill-humour. Unable to comprehend time. Comprehension slow and difficult. Suffers mental torture before and during an electric storm.
- Loss of memory.
- Loss of consciousness.
- Loss of sensibility.
- Dulness of head.
- Stupefaction. Giddiness, especially on stooping.

Head

- Headache; pressure in the forehead, from above downwards, as from a stone.
- Tearing from the nape of the neck to the forehead.
- Painful spasms in the head.
- Sore pain in the occiput.
- Disagreeable shocks, generally in the occiput.
- Roaring in the whole sinciput.
- Feeling of coldness on the vertex.
- The growth of the hair is considerably promoted.

Eyes

- Sensation as if the eyes were deep in the head.
- Sensation as if something would come out of the eyeball.
- Inflammation of the eyes; profuse lachrymation.
- Dim-sightedness.
- Blindness.
- Black point before the right eye.
- Everything looks yellow.

Ears

- Darting in the right ear, from the throat.
- Drawing from the jaws into the ears.
- Swelling of the inner ear.
- Blisters behind the ears full of an acrid fluid.
- Whizzing in the ears, or sensation as if obstructed by a plug.

Nose

- Loss of smell.
- Discharge of a milky fluid from the nose.

Face

- Expression of terror in the countenance.
- Scurf in the face, on the arms and body.
- Large blisters on the cheeks.

Teeth

- Tearing in the upper teeth, proceeding from the head.
- Pain as from subcutaneous, ulceration in old sockets of the molar teeth.

Mouth and Pharynx

- Increased secretion of saliva.
- Foam at the mouth.
- The tongue is very sensitive, particularly at the tip.
- Swelling of the tongue.

Throat

- Loss of speech, inability to articulate.
- Blisters on the palate, the epidermis becoming detached.
- Constant titilation in the throat.
- Inflammation of the pharynx.

Gastro-intestinal System

- Heartburn.
- Ptyalism.
- Nausea, also after a meal.
- Desire to vomit.
- Vomiting with sore throat.
- Haematemesis.
- Sense of repletion in the stomach, after a slight meal.
- Cutting in the abdomen at the approach of a thunderstorm.
- Black-yellow, liquid stools, having a foetid smell.
- Drawing up of the testes during stool.
- Violent pressing in the anus (during menses).
- Burning at the anus.
- Flowing haemorrhoids.

Urinary System

- Frequent micturition.
- Incontinence of urine.
- Discharge of blood with the urine.

Female Reproductive System

- Appearance of the menses (while in the electric bath).
- Black and thick menstrual blood.
- Profuse menses, with pressing in rectum.
- Leucorrhoea, first thin, then thick, with coagula of the size of a hazel nut.

Larynx and Trachea

- Cough with violent titilation in the throat and pressure in the forehead from within outward.

Respiration

- Asthma all one's life, with palpitation of the heart and disposition to faint.

Chest

- Palpitation of the heart, with fever, or with headache or with oppressive anxiety and bright-red face.
- Chest and arms become stiff, almost paralyzed : unable to walk.
- Heaviness and stiffness of chest and shoulders, felt like marble.

Back

- Boils in the back and nape of the neck.
- Stinging in a swollen cervical gland.

Upper Limbs

- Frightful pains in the arms and lower limbs.
- Paralysis of the arms.
- Trembling of the hands.
- Swelling of the hand, also red, or sudden.
- Feeling of numbness in the tips of the fingers.
- Blister filled with a greenish, sanguinous fluid on the finger which discharges the blood.

Lower Limbs

- Burning in the foot, up to the knees, particularly at night.
- Coldness of the lower extremities up to the abdomen, in summer, during a cool wind.
- Tingling in the soles of the feet. Sensation as of a broad ring around the malleoli.
- Intense suffering of electric shocks through left foot and entire 1- side of body to head, repeated at every discharge during a thunder-storm.

Sleep

- Yawning, with shuddering over the whole body.
- Sleeplessness for two months.

Fever

- Shuddering over the body, every morning with yawning.
- Chilliness, then dry, short heat.
- Frequent alternation of chilliness and heat, with sore throat.
- Chilliness with profuse sweat, with painful spasms in the head and along the back.
- Excessive night sweat in an arthritic individual, without relief; sweat with anxiety during a thunder-storm.

Skin

- Violent pains and swelling of the foot which had been frozen twelve years ago.
- Red pimples on the spot touched by the sparks.
- White vesicles.
- The skin becomes blackish.
- Ecchymosis.

General Symptoms

- Pains in the limbs.
- Drawing through all the limbs, extending to the tips of the fingers and toes.
- Shock through the whole body, proceeding from the malar bone.
- Tingling in the electrified parts.
- Violent burning of the parts which are in contact with the chain.
- General languor after a meal.

- Relaxation of the nerves and muscles.
- Fainting.
- Stiffness of the limbs.
- Paralysis of single limbs, particularly the lower.
- Trembling of the limbs, particularly of those which have received the shock.
- Subsultus tendinum.
- Painful spasms along the back from below upward.
- St. Vitus' dance.
- Aggravation of epileptic fits.
- Intense suffering with paralysis of nervous and muscular system.
- Heavy sensation as if she weighed a ton.

LAC FELINUM
(Cat's Milk)

Mental Generals

- Great depression of spirits.
- Very cross to every one.
- Fear of falling downstairs, but without vertigo.
- Mental illusion that the corners of furniture, or any pointed object near her, were about to run into eyes; the symptom is purely mental; the objects do not appear to her sight to be too close (asthenopia).

Head

- Dull pain in forehead in region of eye brows.
- Actual pains on vertex.
- Actual pain over l.eye and temple.

- Pain in head < from reading.
- Pain in forehead, occiput, and 1.side of head, with rigidity of cords of neck (splenius and trapezius), and heat in vertex; the pain in forehead is heavy pressing down over eyes (headache).
- Intense pain from head along lower jaw, causing mouth to fill with saliva.
- Crawling on top of brain (asthenopia).
- Weight on vertex (asthenopia).
- Terrible headache penetrating 1. eyeball to centre of brain, with pain in 1. supra-orbital region extending through brain to vertex (headache).
- Burning on 1. temple near eye, < at night (keratitis).

Eyes

- Sharp lancinating pain through centre of 1. eyeball leaving it very sore internally, and causing profuse lachrymation (from the 1 m).
- Heavy pressure downwards of eyebrows and eyelids, as if the parts were lead.
- Inclination to keep eyes shut.
- On looking fixedly, reading, or writing, darting pain from eyes nearly to occiput; much < in r. eye (asthenopia).
- When reading letters run together, with dull aching pain behind eyes, or shooting in eyes, the confused sight and shooting being < in r. eye; symptoms excited by catching cold or by over-fatigue (asthenopia).
- Pain in eyes, back into head, extremely sharp, with a sensation as if eyes extended back; great photophobia to natural or artificial light; any continued glare results in this pain (improved).
- Photophobia.

- Stye on l. upper lid.
- Eyes get bad every September.
- Eyes ache by gaslight.
- A black spot before r. eye. moving with the eye when in sunlight.
- Sensation of sand in r. eye on walking.

Have had great success with it in eye cases, esp. where there is severe pain in back of orbit, indicating choroidits - Swan

Teeth
- Pain in all the teeth as the hot pain from head touched them.

Mouth
- Sensation as if tongue were scale by a hot drink.
- Redness under tongue, on gums, and whole buccal cavity.
- Loss of taste.
- Brassy taste in mouth.
- Salivation, tongue enlarged and serrated at edges by teeth.
- Very sore mouth.

Throat
- Tough mucus in pharynx.
- Stringy, tough mucus in pharynx, cannot hawk it up and has to swallow it; when it can be expectorated it is yellow.
- Posterior wall of pharynx slightly inflamed, with sensation of soreness.

Respiratory System

- dryness of rim of glottis.

Chest

- Very much oppressed for breath, continuing for several days; it is a difficulty in drawing a long breath, or rather that requires the drawing of a long inspiration, for it seems as if the breathing was done by upper part of lungs alone.

Gastro-intestinal System

- No appetite,
- Great desire to eat paper.
- Stomach sore all around just below the belt, < l. side.
- Heat in epigastrium.
- Great soreness and sensitiveness of epigastric regions.
- Pain in abdomen and back, as if menses are about commencing.
- Great weight and bearing down in pelvis, like falling of the womb, as if she could not walk; < when standing.
- Pain in pelvis through hips on pressure, as when placing arms akimbo.
- Natural stool, but very slow in passing, at 2 A.M.
- Stool long, tenacious, slipping back when ceasing to strain; seeming inability of rectum to expel it its contents.

Urinary System

- Frequent desire to urinate, urine very pale.
- Obstruction in urinating, has to wait.

Female Reproductive System

- leucorrhoea ceased on third day and reappeared on fourth day.

- Furious itching of vulva, inside and out; yellow leucorrhea.
- Dragging pain in left ovary.

Upper Limbs

- Pain in r. side of l. wrist when using index finger.

Lower Limbs

- L. foot feel cold when touched by r. foot Legs ache.

Sleep

- Dullness, sleepiness, gaping.
- Heavy, profound sleep, not easily awakened.

Fever

- Cold and heat alternately, each continuing but a short time.

Generalities

- Entire r. side from crown to sole felt terribly weak, heavy, and distressed, so that it was difficult to walk.
- Constant nervous trembling, esp. of hands, as in drunkards.

LAC VACCINUM

(Cow's Milk)

Mental Generals

- General nervousness, with depression of spirits, feeling as though about to hear bad news.
- Mental confusion, lasting a long time after proving.
- Mental prostration, came on so suddenly, was unable to collect her thoughts or write her symptoms.

Head

- Vertigo : falls backwards if she closes her eyes.
- Fulness of head as it too large and heavy.
- Vertigo.

Eyes

- Dull pain over r. eye, and very slight dull feeling over l. eye.
- Eyes have a blur, or dimness, or obscurity of sight, off and on for a few moments at a time.

Ears

- Ears felt stopped up; felt deaf in both ears, although she could hear as before.

Mouth

- Had a dirty, yellow-coated tongue, which felt parched.
- Sour taste.
- Acid saliva staining handkerchief yellow.
- Ulcers on tongue, flat, white, sunken; tongue swollen, exceedingly sensitive, covered with white, slimy mucus on the parts not ulcerated; breath extremely foetid; sores extend to inside cheeks and tonsils; deglutition painful.

Throat

- Sensation of plug in throat or larynx.

Respiratory System

- Sensation of plug in throat or larynx.

Appetite

- Thirst for cold water in quantities; drank three tumblerfuls during evening.

Gastro-intestinal System

- Had a swelling or bloating of stomach (3d).

- At 10.30 A.M. sour taste, nausea, but no rising or vomting (1 h).
- Eructations.
- Pain proceeding from sternum, extending across abdomen about an inch below umbilicus.
- Constant intolerable flatulence, begins an hour after drinking milk for lunch and lasts all the afternoon.
- Borborygmus, with loud, noisy rumbling (200).
- Obstinate constipation; stool hard, dry; in impacted balls; can be passed only with great straining.
- Passage of stinking flatus, in large quantity, which relieves.

Female Reproductive System
- White watery leucorrhoea; pain in sacrum.
- Drinking a glass of milk will promptly suppress the flow until next menstural period.
- Menses, suppressed, delayed by putting hands in cold water.
- "Nausea of pregnancy with desire for food > by drinking milk."

Back
- Pains in sacrum.

Lower Limbs
- Piercing or lancinating pain in each hip joint, not severe.
- Short rheumatic pains in knee and tarsal joints when walking.

Skin
- Brown crusts, having a greasy appearance, especially in corners of mouth, similar to what are called "butter-sores."

Generalities

- The pains in chest, abdomen, hips, thighs, and knees were all felt on r. and l. sides simultaneously.

MAGNETIS POLI AMBO

(The Magnet)

Mental Generals

- While attending to his business in the day-time, he talks aloud to himself, without being aware of it.

- Excessive exhaustion of the body, with feeling of heat, and cool sweat in the face with unceasing and, as it were, hurried and overstrained activity.

- Hurried headlessness and forgetfulness; he says and does something different from what he intends, omitting letters, syllables and words.

- He endeavours to do things, and actually does thing contrary to his own intentions.

- Wavering, irresolutiness, hurriedness.

- He is unable to fix his attention on one object.

- The things around him strike him like one who is half dreaming.

- He inclines to be angry and vehement; and after he has become angry, his head aches as if sore.

- He is disposed to feel vexed; this gives him pain, especially a headache, as if a nail were forced into his head.

Sensorium

- Vertigo in the evening after lying down, as if he would fall, or resembling a sudden jerk through the head.

- When walking he staggers from time to time, without feeling giddy.
- The objects of sight seem to be wavering, this makes him stagger when walking.

Head

- Whizzing in the whole head, occasioned by the imposition of magnetic surfaces on the thighs, legs and chest.
- The head feels confused as when one takes opium.
- When endeavouring to think of something and fatiguing his memory, he is attached with headache.
- Headache, as is felt after catching cold.
- Headache occasioned by the least chagrin, as if a sharp pressure were made on a small spot in the brain.
- Pain in the region of the vertex, at a small spot in the brain, as if a blunt nail were pressed into the brain; the spot feels sore to the touch.
- Sensation on top of the head, as if the head and the whole body were pressed down.

Face

- Cold hands, with heat in the face and smarting sensation in the skin of the face.
- Intolerable burning prickings in the muscles of the face, in the evening.
- Sweat in the face without heat, early in the morning.

Eyes

- Dilated pupils with cheerfulness of the mind and body.
- Fiery sparks before the eyes, like shooting stars.
- Sensation in the eye as if the pendulum of a clock were moving in it.
- White, luminous, sudden vibrations, like reflections of light, at twilight, on one side of the visual ray, all round.

- Itching of the eyelids and eyeballs in the inner canthus.
- Sensation as if the eyelids were dry.
- Twitching of the lower eyelid.

Ears

- Fine whistling in the ear, coming and going like the pulse.
- Whizzing before the ears.
- Electric shocks in the ear.
- Hard hearing without noise in the ear.

Nose

- Illusion of smell : smell of manure before the nose, from time to time he imagines he has a smell before the nose such as usually comes out of a chest full of clothes which had been closed for a long while.

Teeth and Jaws

- Metallic taste on one side of the tongue.
- Tearing pain in the periosteum of the upper jaw, coming with a jerk and extending as far as the orbit; the pain consists in a tearing, boring, pricking and burning.
- Darting-tearing pain in the facial bones, especially the antrum Highmorianum. in the evening.
- When taking a cold drink, the coldness rushes into the teeth.
- Looseness of the teeth.
- Toothache, excited by stooping.
- The gums of a hollow tooth are swollen and painful to the touch.
- Aching pain of the hollow, carious, teeth.
- Uniform pain in the roots of the lower incisors, as if the teeth were bruised, sore or corroded.

Mouth and Pharynx

- Shocks in the jaws.
- Pain of the submaxillary gland as if swollen, early in the morning in open air.
- Ptyalism every evening with swollen lips.
- Bad smell from the mouth which he does not preceive himself also with much mucus in the throat.
- Continual foetid odour from the mouth, without himself perceiving it, as in incipient mercurial ptyalism.
- Burning of the tongue, and pain of the same when eating.

Taste and Appetite

- Hunger, especially in the evening.
- He has an appetite, but the food has no taste.
- He has a desire for tobacco, milk, beer, and he relishes those things; but he feels satisfied immediately after commencing eating.
- Aversion to tobacco, although he relished it.
- Want of appetite without any loathing, repletion or bad smell.

Gastro-intestinal System

- Eructations, tasting and smelling like the dust of sawed or turned horn.
- The erucations taste of the ingesta, but as if spoiled.
- Crackling and cracking in the pit of the stomach, as when a clock is wound up.
- Sensation of an agreeable distension in the region of the diaphragm.
- Pressure in the epigastrium, as from a stone, especially when reflecting much.
- Tensive aching and anxious repletion in the epigastrium.

- The flatulence moves about in the abdomen, with loud rumbling, painless incarceration of flatulence in various small places of the abdomen, causing a sharp aching pain and an audible grunting.

- Loud, although painless rumbling, especially in the lesser intestines, extending under the public bones and into the groin, as if diarrhoea would come on.

- Emission of short and broken flatulence, with loud noise and pains in the anus.

- Loud rumbling in the abdomen, early in the morning when in bed; afterwards colic as if from incarceration of flatulence.

- Putrid fermentation in the bowels, the flatulence has a foetid smell and is very hot.

- Qualmish sensation and painfulness in the intestines, as if one had taken a resinous cathartic or rhubarb, with painful emission of hot, putrid flatulence.

- Every emission of flatulence is preceded by pinching in the abdomen.

- Tensive and burning pain in the epigastrium and hypogastrium, followed by a drawing and tensive pain in the calves.

- Itching of the umbilicus.

- Diarrhoea without colic

- Constipation as if the rectum were constricted and contracted.

- Violent haemorrhoidal pain in the anus after stool, erosive as if sore, and as if the rectum were constricted.

- Burning at the anus when sitting, as in haemorrhoids.

- Itching haemorrhoids.

- Blind haemorrhoids after soft stool, as if the varices on

the margin of the anus felt sore, both when sitting and walking.

- Prolapsus recti when going to stool.

Urinary System

- Burning in the bladder, especially in the region of the neck of the bladder, a few minutes after urinating.

Male Sexual System

- Burning in the urethra, in the region of the caput gallinaginis, during an emission of semen.
- Early in the morning he feels a burning in the region of the vesiculae seminales.
- Nightly emissions of semen.
- Violent continuous erections, early in the morning when in bed, without any sexual desire.
- Want of sexual desire, aversion to an embrace.
- The penis remains in a relaxed condition, in spite of all sexual excitement.
- The prepuce retreats entirely behind the glans.
- Swelling of the epididymis, with simple pain when feeling it or during motion.
- Itching smarting of the inner surface of the prepuce.
- Menses had ceased a few days before, returned next day after imposing the magnetic surface and continued ten days.

Larynx

- Frequent fits of nightly cough which does not wake him.
- Convulsive cough.
- Mucus in the trachea which is easily hawked up, evening and morning.
- Violent fit of cough, with profuse expectoration of blood.

Chest and Lungs

- Asthma after midnight when waking and reflecting, occasioned by mucus in the chest, diminished by coughing.
- Spasmodic cough, with shocks in the chest and anxious breathing, and visible oppression of the chest.
- Violent oppression of the chest, tearing in the stomach and bowels, and beating in the shoulders.

Back

- Painful stiffness of the cervical vertebra in the morning, during motion.
- Crackling in the cervical vertebra in the morning during motion.
- Pain in the omo-hyoid muscle, as if it would be attached with cramp.
- Pain in the back when standing or sitting quiet.
- Burning in the dorsal spine.
- Twitching of the muscles of the back and sensation as if something were alive in them.
- Pain in sacro-lumbar articulation, in the morning when in bed lying on the side, and in day-time when stooping a long time.
- Shock or jerk in the small of the back, almost arresting the breathing.

Upper Limbs

- Tearing jerkings in the muscles of the arm when staying in a cold place.
- Shocks in the top of the shoulder which caused the arms to recede from the body with a jerk.
- Shocks in the arm-joints and head, as if those parts were beaten with a light and small hammer.
- Prickings in the arm.

- Beating and throbbing in all the joints of the arms and fingers.
- Deep-seated pain in the arm, extending as far as the elbow, the arm going to sleep and trembling spasmodically.
- Drawing from the head down to the tip of the fingers.
- The hands are icy cold the whole day, for several days, from touching the centre of the bar.
- Pain in the wrist-joint, as if a tendon had become strained, or as if an electric shock were passing through the parts.

Lower Limbs

- Attacks of cramp in the calves and toes after walking.
- Drawing from the hips to the feet, leaving a burning along that tract.
- Violent shocks of the right lower limb, occasioned by a burning emanation from the chin and neck through the right side.
- Fiery burning in the upper and lower limbs; when the right limb touched the left one, it seemed as if the latter were set on the fire by the former.
- Pain in the upper part of the tarsal joints, as if the shoe had pinched him, and as if a corn were there.

Sleep

- Coma vigil early in the morning for several hours : after sunrise, sopor or deep sleep set in full of heavy, passionate dreams, for instance, vexing dreams; the sopor terminates in a headache as if the brain were sore all over, disappearing after rising.
- Lascivious dreams, even during the siesta, with discharge of the prostatic fluid.

Skin

- The recent wound commences to bleed again.
- The wound, which is almost healed, commences to pain again like a recent wound.
- Boils break out on various parts of the body, passing of soon.
- Corrosive pain in various parts, for example, below the ankle.

General Symptoms

- Dull, numb pain.
- Jerking shock, causing the trunk to bend violently upward and forward as low down as the hips, with cries.
- Fits of fainting, palpitation of the heart and suffocation.
- Long-lasting swoons, in which she retained her consciousness.

MAGNETIS POLUS ARCTICUS

(North-pole of the Magnet)

Mental Generals

- Out of humour and weary.
- Weeping mood with chilliness and a disposition to feel chilly.
- Sadness, in the evening; he made to weep, contrary to his will, after which his eyes felt sore.
- Indolent fancy; he sometimes felt as if he had no fancy at all.
- Indolent mind.
- While attending to his business, he talks aloud to himself.

- He makes mistakes easily in writing.
- Hasty, bold, quick, firm.
- Calm, composed mood, devoid of care.

Sensorium

- Vertigo, sensation as if she would fall in every direction.
- Vertiginous motion in one side of the head.
- Dullness of the head with desire for open air.
- Weak memory, but he feels cheerful.

Head

- Headache, constucting in a sore and bruised pain in the surface of the brain, in the sinciput and in one of the temples.
- Sensation as if the head were pressed down by a load.
- Disagreeable, compressive sensation in the head, and as if one part of the brain were pressed in.
- Headache, as if the temples were pressed as under.
- Violent headache the whole afternoon, as if the brain were pressed as under.
- Rush of blood to the head, and suffusion of heat in the cheeks.
- Drawing-boring pain in the right temple, accompained with a spasmodic pain below the right malar bone.
- Aching pain over the left temporal region, externally.
- Pushing tearing in the head behind the left ear when sitting.

Eyes

- Cold movement as of a cold breath in th eyes.
- The eyes protrude.
- Staring look.

- Itching in the inner canthus and in the margin of the eye-lids.
- Painful feeling of dryness in the eyelids in the morning on waking.
- Jerking and drawing in the eyelids.
- Drawing in the eyelids with lachrymation.
- Pricking in the eyelids.
- Lachrymation early in the morning.
- Excessive lachrymation; the light of the sun is intolerable.
- Burning in the weak right eye; it became red and filled with water (the magnet being held in contact with the weak right eye for a quarter of an hour).
- Coldness in the weak eye for three or four minutes (the magnet being held in contact with that eye for 2 minutes).
- Uneasy motion of the eye, with a good deal of water accumulating in either eye.
- Sensation as of a cobweb in front of the eyes.
- Formication between the two eyes.
- Strong drawing over the eye, in the surface of the cheek, ear, extending into the upper maxillary bone (the magnet being in contact with the eye).

Nose

- Illusion of smell : he imagines the room smelled of fresh whitewash and dust, he imagines the room smells of rotten eggs, or of the contents of a privy.
- Violent bleeding at the nose, for three afternoons in succession, increasing every afternoon, and preceded by an aching pain in the forehead.
- Redness and heat of the tip of the nose, followed by hot, red circumscribed spots on the cheeks.

Ears
- Fine ringing in the opposite ear (immediately).
- Whizzing an a drawing sensation in the ear.
- Ringing in the ear of same side.
- A kind of deafness, as if a pellicle had been drawn over the right ear, after which heat is felt in the ear.

Face
- Intensely painful tightness in the face, extending as far as the tonsils.
- Drawing in the left cheek.

Jaws and Teeth
- Drawing-aching pain coming from the temple, below the mastoid process, between the sterno-cleido-mastoideus muscle and the ramus of the lower jaw.
- Toothache as if the tooth would be torn out, worse after a meal, and when sitting or lying down, improving when walking.
- Toothache in the direction of the eye, a very quick succession of pecking in the hollow tooth, with swollen inflamed gums and a burning cheek : the toothache increased very much immediately after a meal, improved when walking in the open air, but aggravated in a smoky room.
- Throbbing in the hollow tooth (immediately), followed by a pressure in the tooth as if something had got into the tooth, with drawing in the temples.
- Throbbing in the tooth, with burning in the gums, and swollen, hot cheeks, with burning pain and heat in the cheeks, in the afternoon.
- The toothache ceases when walking in the open air, and returns in the room.

- Aching in the hollow teeth, with swelling of one side of the face.
- Toothache with jerks through the periosteum of the jaw, the pain being a darting-aching, digging-tearing, or burning-stinging pain.
- The toothache is worse after eating and in the warm room.
- Numbness and insensibility of the gums of the painful tooth.
- Drawing pain in the hollow tooth,and fore teeth, increased by anything warm; with redness of the cheek during the pain.
- Swelling of the gums of a hollow tooth, painful when touched with the tongue.
- Toothache, as if the gums were sore or cut, increased by the air entering the mouth.

Mouth

- Sore pain in the left corner of the mouth, when moving it, as if an ulcer would form.
- Painful humming in the hollow teeth of the lower jaw, worse on the right side, the toothache ceases during eating.

Appetite and Taste

- Sourish taste in the morning, as if one were fasting.
- Greedy appetite at supper.

Gastro-intestinal System

- Frequent eructation of mere air.
- Drawing in the pit of the stomach, extending into the right chest.
- Spasmodic contractive sensation in the hypogastrium, externally and internally, early in the morning.

- Flatulent colic immediately after supper ; sharp pressure in every part of the abdomen from within outward, as if the abdomen would burst ; relieved when sitting perfectly still.

- Flatulent colic early in the morning, immediately after, waking ; the flatulence was pressed upward toward the hypochondriac region, with tensive pains in the whole abdomen, causing a hard presure here and there, accompanied with a qualmishness and nausea which proceeded from the abdomen, and was felt both in motion and when at rest.

- Gurgling in the abdomen as if a quantity of flatulence were incarcerated, causing a writhing sensation, which rises up to the pit of the stomach, and causes eructations.

- Relaxed condition of the abdominal ring, increasing from day to day ; hernia threatens to protrude, especially when coughing.

- Sore pain in the abdominal ring, when walking.

- Boring pain above the left abdominal ring, from within outward, as if hernia would protrude.

- Inguinal hernia.

- Drawing, almost dysenteric pain in the hypogastrium, early in the morning, followed by difficult expulsion of the very thick faeces.

- Stinging-pinching in the rectum.

Respiratory System

- Dry cough causing a painful rawness in the chest, especially in the night after getting warm in bed, having been chilly first.

- Racking and spasmodic cough while falling asleep, hindering sleep.

- Suffocative, spasmodic cough about midnight.

Chest
- Pressure in the region of the heart (immediately).
- When walking in the open air he imagines that heat is entering chest, passing through the pharynx.

Sexual System
- Nightly involuntary emission.

Back
- Crackling or cracking in the cervical vertebrae especially in the atlas, during motion.
- Pain as if bruised in the middle of the spine, when bending the spine backward.
- Gurgling and creeping sensation between the scapulae.
- Twitching in the posterior lumbar muscles.
- Pain as if bruised in the left shoulder joint both during motion and rest, painless when touching it.

Upper Extremities
- Cramp-like sensation in the arm, and as if it had gone to sleep.
- Violent coldness in the arm over which the magnet had been moved (in a female in magetic sleep, after being touched with the north-pole magnet).
- Prickling pain in the arm as far as the shoulder, especially in the long bones of the forearm.
- Sore pain in the right shoulder when walking in the open air.
- Stiffness and rigidity in the right tarsal and carpal joints, at night when in bed.
- Painful and almost burning itching in dorsum of the middle phalanx of the little finger, as if the part had been frozen ; the place was painful to the touch.

Lower Extremities

- Tearing with pressure in the outer side of the knees down to the outer ankle.
- Excessive weakness of the lower limbs, when walking, as if they would break.
- Rigid tension in the hamstrings when rising from a seat, as if too short.
- Sore pressure in the corns, which had been painless heretofore, when pressing the feet ever so little.
- Sudden lancinations in the heels, big toe and calf when sitting.
- Painful crawling in the toes of the right foot.

Sleep

- Constant drowsiness in the day-time.
- Lascivious dreams the whole night.
- She saw a person in a dream, and next day she saw that person in reality for the first time.
- Restless sleep ; he tosses about and his bed feels too warm.

Fever

- Sensation of coldness or coolness over the whole body as if she were dressed too lightly, or as if she had taken cold, without shuddering; immediately after she had a small loose stool which was succeeded by pressing.
- Shuddering all over at the moment when the north pole Was touched by the tip of the tongue.
- Cool sweat all over.
- Heat in one of the cheeks, accompanied with a feeling of internal heat, irritable disposition and talkativeness.

Skin

- Crawling over the skin.

General symptoms

- Continuous digging-up stitches in various parts, becoming sharper and more painful, in proportion as they penetrate more deeply into the flesh.
- Tensive sensation in the adjoining parts.
- Bruised pain in the adjoining parts, and as if one had carried a heavy burden.
- Tremulousness through the whole body, especially in the feet.
- Tremor in the part touched by the magnet (immediately).
- Nervousness with trembling, uneasiness in the limbs, great distension of the abdomen, anxiety, solitude and great nervous weakness.
- Sensation of coldness in the part which was touched by the magnet.
- Drawing in the periosteum of all the bones, as is felt at the commencement of an intermittent fever (but without chilliness of heat).
- The faintness, the bruised and painful sensation in the limbs were worse in the open air.

MAGNETIS POLUS AUSTRALIS

(South-pole of the Magnet)

Mental Generals

- Want of cheerfulness : he is low-sprited, as if he were alone, or as if he had experienced some sad event, for three hours.

- Weeping immediately.
- Despondency (the first hours).
- Great discouragement, dissatisfaction with himself.
- Want of disposition to work and vexed mood.
- Taciturn, he is not disposed to talk.
- He wants to be alone, company is disagreeable to him.
- Violent anger excited by a slight cause ; he becomes trembling and hurried, and uses violent language.
- Wild, vehement, rude, both in language and action (he does not perceive it himself) : he asserts with violence, reviling others with distorted countenance.
- Great quickness of fancy.
- Unsteadiness of the mind ; he is unable to fix his ideas ; things seem to flit to and fro before his senses ; his opinions and resolutions are wavering, which occasions a kind of anxious and uneasy condition of the mind.
- Vertigo as if intoxicated, as if he were obliged to stagger, some vertigo even while sitting.

Head

- Rush of blood to the head, without heat.
- Heaviness of the head, with a sort of creeping or fine digging in the head.
- Fine crawling in the brain as of a number of insects, accompained with heaviness of the head.
- Drawing-tearing pain in the left brain, resembling a slow, burning stitch.
- Pressure in the occiput, in alternate places.
- Headache in the occiput, most violent in the room, but disappearing in the open air (in the first hours).
- Spasmodic contractive headache in the region between the eyebrows.

- The skin on the forehead feels as if dried fast to the skull.

Face

- Sensation in the face (and in the rest of the body) as if cold air were blowing upon it.

Eyes

- Watery eyes from time to time.
- Painful, smarting dryness of the eyelids, especially perceptible when moving them mostly in the evening and morning.
- Deficient sight : things looked dim, also double, when touching the nape of the neck.

Ears

- Tearing pains in the cartilages of the outer and inner ear, extending very nearly as far as the inner cavities.
- Roaring in the ears, which he felt more in the upper part of the head.
- Noise in the ears, like the motion of a wing.
- Sensation as of the whizzing of the wind in the ears, early in the morning ; he feels it as far as the forehead.
- Inflammation of the outer ear, the grooves of that portion of the ear assuming the appearance of sore rhagades.
- Occasional stitches and ringing in the ear.

Mouth

- Sensation of swelling in the tongue, and heat in the organs of speech.

Throat

- Burning in the pharynx, a sort of strangulation from below upwards, with a feeling of heat.

Jaws and Teeth

- Toothache, aggravated by warm drink.
- Tearing jerking in the upper jaw towards the eye, in the evening.
- Dull pain with intensely painful stitches in hollow teeth.

Appetite and Taste

- Indifference to milk, bordering on aversion, early in the morning.

Gastro-intestinal System

- Inclination to vomit, early in the morning after waking.
- Fits of nausea when stooping forward, apparently in the stomach.
- Loud rumbling in the abdomen.
- Flatulent colic at night : portions of flatulence seem to spring from one place to another, which is painful, and causes disagreeable grumbling sensation, or a sore pinching pressure from with in outward in many places, depriving him of sleep, short flatus goes off now and then with pain, but affords no relief.
- Drawing pain in the right side of the abdomen, scarcely permitting him to walk.
- Tearing colic occasioned by (reading?) and walking, and appeared by sitting, especially in the epigastrium (early in the morning).
- Distended abdomen in the evening immediately before going to bed, with colicky pains.
- Emission of quantity of flatulence.
- Sensation as if the abdominal ring were enlarged, and as if hernia protruded ; every turn of the cough causes a painful dilation of the ring.

- Frequent desire for stool, causing nausea, but she is unable to accomplish anything.
- Continual contraction and constriction of the rectum and anus, permitting scarcely the least flatulence to be emitted.

Urinary System

- Relaxation of the sphincter vesicae (immediately).
- Incontinence of urine.
- Smarting pain in the forepart of the urethra, during the emission of urine, as if the urine were acrid or sour.

Male Sexual System

- Drawing in the spermatic cord, early in the morning when the testicle hanging down, as if pulled or distended ; the testicle is even painful to the touch.
- Jerking in the spermatic cord.
- Slow, fine, painful drawing in the spermatic cord.
- Tearing in the spermatic cord.
- Spasmodic drawing up of the testicles, in the night.
- Pain in the penis, as if several fleshy fibres were torn or pulled backwards.
- Red spot, like a pimple, on the corona glandis and on the internal surface of the prepuce, without sensation.
- The glans is red and inflamed, with itching and tension.
- Nocturnal emission (in a person affected with hemiplegia) : it had not taken place for years past. (Note by *Hahnemann*-After this emission the paralysis became worse : the sick limb seemed dead to him).
- **Impotence :embrace with the proper sensations and erection : but at the moment when the semen is about to be emitted, the voluptuous sensation is suddenly arrested,**

the semen is not emitted ; and the penis becomes relaxed.

Female Reproductive System

- The menses, which had already lasted the usual time,
continue to flow for six days longer, only during motion,
not when at rest ; every discharge of blood is
accompained with a cutting pain in the abdomen. (Note
by *Hahenmann.*This woman held the south-pole, touching at the same time the middle of the bar. The south-
pole appears to excite haemorrhage and especially from
the uterus, as its primary effect ; the north-pole seems to
act in the contrary manner.)
- The menses, which were to appear in a few days, appeared four hours after the south-pole had been touched,
but the blood was light-coloured and watery.

Respiratory System

- Shortness of breath in the pit of the stomach.

Chest

- Palpitation of the heart.

Back

- Gnawing and smarting in the back.

Upper Extremities

- Crawling in the left arm, from above downward, resem-
bling small snakes.
- Quick, painful jerking, in the arms, from above down-
ward.
- Jerking in the fingers which are touched by the magnet.
- Sense of heat and jerking in the finger touching the mag-
net.
- Beating in the finger in contact with magnet.

Lower Extremities

- Drawing, with pressure, in the muscles of the thighs, worse during motion.
- Sense of coldness in the right thigh.
- Drawing pain in the outer side of the bend of the knee.
- Tearing with pressure in the patella (worse during motion), and aggravated by feeling the part.
- Cracking of the knee-joint during motion.
- Itching-burning, slow stitch in the side of the calf.
- Soreness of the inner side of the nail of the big toe in the flesh, as if the nail had grown into the flesh on one side ; very painful, even when slightly touched.
- Pinching occasioned by the shoes on top and on the sides of the toes, and near the nail of the big toe when walking, as from corns.

Sleep

- Frequent yawning (With chilliness).
- Sleepless and wakeful before midnight, and no disposition to go to sleep.
- Restless, frequently turns from side to side, in the night when in bed.
- Dreams about fires.
- He quarrels and fights in a dream.
- Unusual beating in the region of the heart.

Fever

- Chills in the room the whole day, especially after an evening nap.
- Chilliness of the legs upto the knee, with a sensation of heat and blood to the heat.
- Feeling of coldness all over, in the evening (without shud-

dering), without thirst (except at the commencement of the chilliness), and without being actually cold ; at the same time he feels out of humour, everything was disagreeable to him, even the meal, two hours after he was covered with heat and sweat all over, without thirst.

- During the chilliness, or the feeling of coldness, he was quite warm, but he was obliged to lie down, and to cover himself well ; his mouth was very dry ; afterwards he was covered with a profuse sweat all over, without feeling hot ; on the contrary, he felt a constant shuddering over the perspiring parts, as if they were covered with goose-skin ; accompanied with a sensation as of a breeze blowing into the ears.

- Warmth all over, especially in the back.

Skin

- Corrosive itching in the evening, when in bed, on the back and other parts of the body.

- Itching, stinging, tearing, here or there, in the evening, when in bed.

General Symptoms

- Bruised pain in all the limbs, so that he imagined he was lying on stones, on whatsoever side of the body he lay.

- Stiffness of the joints.

- Lightness of the whole body.

- Laziness and heaviness of the whole body, accompanied with a feeling of anxiety, as if he were threatened with paralysis, and as if he would fall, accompanied with a feeling of heat in the face and the whole body, mingled with shuddering.

MALANDRINUM

(The Grease of Horses)

Mental Generals

- Confusion and lassitude of the mental faculties with a dread of any mental exertion and a lack of concentration, an entirely new and unusual experience which continued several weeks after stopping the remedy.
- Comprehension difficult.
- Memory weakened and impaired ; great difficulty in remembering what was read.
- Sharp darting pain first in left temple then in right. Confusion and lassitude of mental faculties ; lack of concentration and a dread of any mental exertion.
- Melancholy with general fatigue.

Head

- Pustular eruption on scalp. Sensation of weariness at junction of atlas with cranium, every morning on rising.
- Itching on scalp, especially in the evening.
- Excessive oily dandruff (an entirely new experience) the fourth week after pustules dried up.
- Impetigo covering head from crown to neck and extending behind ears.
- Impetigo, covering back of head, extending over back to buttocks, labia and even into vagina.
- Frontal and occipital headache, backache, weariness and chilliness, lasting one day.
- Frontal headache. on appetite, bilious vomiting and weariness.
- Dizziness.
- Frontal headache. dizziness, backache.

- Temporal headache, dizziness, backache.
- Terrible headache, bone pains, vomiting (bilious), chilliness, diarrhoea, malaise.
- Heaviness in the head.
- Headache and backache, stiffness of neck, loss of appetite, constipation, and great weakness (following vaccination).
- Eruption on forehead, crusty with intense itching.

Face

- Eczema facialis ; intense burning, much oedema, oozing viscid fluid.
- A yellowish honey-comb crust on upper lip.

Ears

- Profuse purulent, greenish yellow discharge, mixed with blood.

Mouth

- Tongue, coated yellow ; with red streak through middle, cracked and ulcerating down middle; swollen.
- Horribly offensive breath.
- Canker on left border of tongue, which spreads in all directions ; tongue sore, unable to speak.
- In one case in which I was using Malandrinum 30 as a prophylactic of variola, it cured a very stubborn case of aphthae *H.S. Taylor*.

Throat

- Sore and swollen < left side. Left tonsil swollen;yellow ulcer with clear cut, well defined edges persistent for several days ; rough scraping sensation like a corn husk or a foreign body, which must be removed mechanically; painless swallowing.

- Left tonsil swollen and inflamed.
- Throat symptoms and pains in throat begin on left side, and extend to right.
- Ulcerated sore throat and tendency to extend downward, invading the larynx.

Throat

- Thirstless ; water nauseates.

Teeth and Gums

- Gums swollen, ulcerate, receding from teeth : bleed easily when touched ; unable to brush the teeth from teeth: bleed easily when touched ; unable to brush the teeth from sore and bleeding gums.
- A dark, brown, tenacious mucus mixed with blood and pus exudes from ulcerated gums.
- Sordes on the teeth.

Gastro-intestinal System

- Nausea after eating ; vomiting of bilious matter.
- Empty, faint, "all gone"sensation, with faintness and trembling, not > by eating, though desire for food is very marked.
- Pains around umbilicus.
- Diarrhoea ; yellow, bloody, slimy ; very changeable, worse in the morning ; acrid, excoriating; child had a dried-up mummyfied appearance ; sleepless and has not nursed for 24 hours.
- Dark, thin, cadaverous-smelling stool.
- Diarrhoea ; acrid, yellow, offensive, followed by burning in anus and rectum.
- Dark brown, foul-somelling, almost involuntary diarrhoea; pains in abdomen.

- Dark brown, painless diarrhoea.
- Black, foul-smelling diarrhoea ; weariness, nausea, dizziness.
- Yellow, foul-smelling, almost involuntary diarrhoea and great weariness.
- Black, foul-smelling, diarrhoea, malaise and weariness.

  Bowels inactive, no desire : move after enema, but leave sore bruised sensation in rectum for hours ; dreads stool.

Urinary System

- Great sensitiveness of bladder on waking ; bladder irritable, frequent desire to urinate.

Male Sexual System

- (Child constantly handles the pains);

Female Reproductive System

- Vagina closed with thick impetiginous crusts ; yellowish, greenish, brown in colour.

Back

- Intense pain across small of back.
- Pain along back as if beaten.
- Backache was intense in the sacral region ; in the dorsal region under the shoulder blades, chiefly the left side ; it was almost unbearable. (Dr. B. from three doses of the 200th).

Upper Limbs

- Impetiginous crusts on extensor sides of forearms. Rhagades in palms and fingers.

Lower Limbs

- Petechia on both thighs < on left.
- Knock-knee.

- Weak ankles, easily turn on making a false step.
- Profuse foot-sweat with carrion-like odour ; toes so sore unable to walk ; only > was when feet were bared and elevated.
- Soles of feet bathed in sweat, scald and burn when covered or warm.
- Large blisters on soles of both feet-no change of shoes-skin exfoliated on both feet.
- Feet "go to sleep" upon least provocation, a sensation never before observed.
- Deep rhagades, sore and bleeding, on soles of feet > in cold weather and after bathing.
- Sore in all limbs and joints.
- "Run arounds" on all nails of hands and feet.

Skin

- Eczema of face and scalp, with burning, stinging itching.
- Impetigo on extensors of forearms.
- Dry, rough, unhealthy skin remaining for years after vaccination.
- Skin rough, dry, harsh.
- Palms and soles thick ; deep rhagades < in cold weather, < from washing with any kind of soap.
- Skin greasy ; oily eruption, and hair excessively oily.
- Pustules slow to develop but never ending ; as one healed another appeared.
- Eruption in hollow of arms and knees, red scaly with intense itching < when becoming warm.

Sleep

- Restless sleep ; dreams of trouble, of quarrels.

- For the bad effects of vaccination has been used with best results.
- When used as a prophylactic for variola has proved protective in many cases, and also prevented vaccination from "taking."
- Lower half of body affected ; greasy skin ; greasy eruption.
- Slow pustulation, never ending, as one healed another appeared.-*Burnett.*

Bad effects of vaccinations ; has cured cases of unhealthy, dry, rough skin, remaining for years after vaccination in small Box, measles and impetigo. - *Clarke.*

- Eczema facialis ; oozing of a viscid fluid ; intense burning, much oedema ; small scales, exfoliated < from bathing at night ; > in cold air.-*Thompson.*
- Impetigo covering back of head, extending over whole back to buttocks and even into vagina, covering labia and extensors of forearms.
- Boils. Malignant pustules.
- *Bad effects of vaccination.*
- Small dusky red spots on legs, not disappearing on pressure.

MALARIA OFFICINALIS

Mental Generals
- Feels stupid and sleepy.
- Very thoughtful.

Head
- Feeling as though he would become dizzy.

- Waving dizziness on falling asleep.
- Dizziness on rising from reclining position.
- Dull aching through forehead and temples.
- Dull headache, dizzy and drowsy.
- Frequent attacks of headache, especially in the forehead.
- Throbbing pain all over head.
- Vertigo ; confused sensation ; worse by walking, turning around, rising or stooping.
- Headache beginning in forehead, extending all over head.

Eyes

- Aching above inner angle of r. eye.
- Eyes feel heavy and sleepy.
- Eyes burn like coals of fire.

Ears

- Drawing pain in r. external ear.

Nose

- A kind of concentration of feeling at root of nose and just above, as though I should have a severe cold like hay-fever.

Face

- Itching on r. cheek over malar bone (and various parts of face and limbs) ; > by slight rubbing or scratching.
- Face becomes warm as if flushed ; and spreads over body.

Respiratory System

- Shallow breathing, which seems from languor, desire to breathe occasionally.
- Residence in malarial districts is said to cure phthisis.
- A consumptive constitution is protected against malaria.

Chest
- Tired feeling through chest and abdomen.
- Constant hacking cough, half minute guns, when talking and turning over in bed.
- Frequent sighing, takes a deep inspiration : restless and nervous.

Mouth
- Pain in upper l. teeth.
- Sensation on point of tongue as if a few specks of pepper were there.
- Saliva more profuse than usual, keeps him swallowing often.
- Tongue coated slightly yellowish-white.
- (Bitter taste, parched mouth ; tongue white.
- Tongue white, with brown streak down the middle.
- Tongue white and thickly coated.
- Mouth very dry, subjectively, but really moist.

Appetite
- Wants cold drinks.
- Cant't eat anything ; vomits everything.
- Craves sour.
- Thirsty ; craves cold water.
- No appetite ; aversion to food, though of it sicken.
- Thirsty for lemonade ; not so much for water.
- Variable ; craves potatoes, apples, beefsteak.
- Bitter, nauseating, bad taste in the mouth.
- Dryness at root of tongue ; buccal cavity seems constricted and contracted.

Gastro-intestinal System

- Unusually hearty appetite (for supper)
- Odour from cooking is pleasing, but no desire for dinner.
- On sitting down eats a good dinner with relish.
- Feels better after eating dinner.
- Easy belching, several times, on taste.
- Qualmish.
- Nausea.
- Retching and gagging from hawking mucus.
- Sense of heat in abdomen.
- Uneasiness in lower abdomen.
- Liver, spleen and kidneys affected.
- Cannot breathe on account of pain in liver, < lying down, > hard pressure.
- Drawing or pricking in liver.
- Cramping in liver, pain under r. scapula.
- Great uneasiness through abdomen, sense of heaviness, Constipation.
- Diarrhoea, no pain ; weakness in bowels.
- Steady, dull pains in region of liver > after urinating.
- Aching under right scapula ; cramp with soreness and sensitiveness in region of liver ; from pressure < by lying down.
- Diarrhoea.
- Diarrhoea in morning, stools thin, yellow, foul.
- Haemorrhoids for many years ; external bleeding ; no pain but very unpleasant.
- Diarrhoea; four or five motions daily of thin, bloody, streaked mucus ; no faecal matter.

Neck and Back

- Neck feels tired, with slight aching in upper parts on moving the head.
- Lumbar region tired as though it would ache.
- Rheumatism of back and limbs, with lameness.
- Stiff neck, and r. arm and shoulders painful and helpless.
- Aching under r. scapula ; cramping in liver.
- Backache in lumbar region, shoots up back: worse when first lying down ; worse after walking ; better lying on the abdomen.

Upper Limbs

- A sense of coldness ascending over body from the legs.
- Gout.
- Limbs get numb and cold.
- Aching in both elbows.
- Aching and tired feeling in wrists ; tired ache in the hands.
- Arms tired.
- Hands seem to be semi-paralyzed, useles, but can use them by force of will.
- Very cold hands during the day ; hands and feet very cold at night.

Lower Limbs

- Pain, upper part of r. illium.
- Tired ache in knees and for some distance above and below.
- Aching in an old (cured) bunion on l. foot.
- Legs restless, feel like stretching and moving them.
- Soles of the feet cold, almost numb.

- Right knee weak and painful, worse when bending, and raising up.

Limbs in General

- Sensation of fatigue in upper extremities first ; later extending to lower extremities and entire system.
- Dull pain in the muscles of the back, lumbar region; uneasy; tired.
- Dull aching pain in left sciatic nerve, and on outer surface of left hip.
- Sensation of burning flush, rising from knees to throat, but without sweat ; relieved by lying down.
- Dull pain in right hip with soreness and tenderness on pressure in the sheaths of the muscles about the hip and tendons of muscles of the thigh.
- Waking at midnight, feet extremely hot with burning palms and soles ; this was followed by profuse sweat on lower part of body, more marked on flexor surfaces and on the back.
- Drawing, shooting pain on left hypochondrium, extending down left leg.
- Arms feel heavy.
- Burning of hands and feet ; aching of hands and arms.

Nerves

- Great reslessness all night, worse towards morning . Could not find a position in which he could rest.

Sleep

- Impelled to lie down, and on falling asleep a sense of waving dizziness passes all over, preventing sleep.
- Gaping, yawning, and desire to stretch.
- Sleep all the time ; can go to sleep while standing.

- Sleepy and drowsy, but sleep does not relieve ; wakes up weary and unrefreshed.

Hypochondria

- Dull throbbing pain in hepatic region for three days, relieved by pressure of corset and by lying on the painful side.

Skin

- Skin, eyes, and face very yellow.
- Skin dry all over ; no sweat at all.

Fever

- Coldness ascending over body from legs.
- A feeling as if he would have a chill, then as if he would become feverish, though neither is very marked.
- Intemittent : quotidian ; tertian (No.II).
- Ague every other day, weak and drowsy between attacks.
- Dumb chills.
- Shooting pains all over in the muscles ; bones ache.
- High fever during night ; also in the morning.
- Chill begins about noon ; every other day. Icy cold from hips down ; chilly all over : fever worse about the trunk. and slight general sweat.
- Aching all over body, especially in arms and legs ; chilly sensation, then breaks out in slight perspiration; frequent recurring attacks.
- Chilly every second day followed by heat ; profuse sweat during the night ; wakes up chilly and takes cold as perspiration ceases.

Generalities

- General sense of weariness ; from a very short walk ;

esp. through pelvis, sacral region, and upper thighs ; strong desire to lie down.

- A kind of simmering all through the body.
- Typhoidal, semi-paralytic condition (No. III).
- Rheumatism.
- Rheumatic paralysis and emaciation.
- Feels very weak and languid ; restless ; does not want to move.
- Great weakness as though he had a long illness, with loss of appetite.
- Great exhaustion.
- Must have doors and windows open ; a close room < head and stomach, and fresh, cool air chills her.

THYROIDIN

Thyriod Extract   *A sarcode*

Trituration of the fresh thyroid gland of sheep or calf. Attenuation of a liquid extract of the gland.

Mental Generals

- Depression.
- Fretfulness and moroseness gave way to cheerfulness and animation.
- Delirium of persecution (three cases observed, one fatal, the result of taking Thyro. in tablets to reduce obesity).
- Sudden acute mania occurring in myxoedema, perfectly restored mentally and bodily under Thyr.
- Mental aberration dating three years before onset of myxoedema subject to attacks of great violence, with

intervals of depression and moroseness.
- State of idiocy ; fearful nightmares.
- Very excited ; excited state followed by considerable depression.
- Irritable and ill-tempered.
- Became a grumbler.
- Angry.
- Had frights.

Head

- Vertigo.
- Feeling of lightness in the brain, scarcely amounting to giddiness.
- Much giddiness and headache for twenty-four hours.
- Awake about 4 A.M. with sharp headache and intense aching in back and limbs, which continued for three days and compelled him to be on his bed.
- Constant headache, pains in occiput and vertex.
- Headache in case of acromegaly.
- Headache.
- In one case of scleroderma and one case of myxoedema the hair fell off permanently.)
- In a case of myxoedema the patient lost all the hair of his head and face and had a thick growth over his arms and thorax; under Thyr. The hair of the head and face grew again and that of the arms and chest fell off.

Eyes

- Prominence of eyeballs-exophthalmic goitre.
- Optic neuritis (in five persons, four of them women, under treatment for obesity ; no other symptoms of thyrodism).
- Accommodative asthenopia.

Ears

- Moist patches behind ears heal up (case of psoriasis). Hyperplastic media otitis with sclerosis and loss of mobility of the ossicles (rapid amelioration-several cases).

Face

- flushing ; with nausea and lumbar pains ; loss of consciousness, tonic muscular spasms ; immediate with rise of temperature, and pains all over ; suddenly became breathless and livid.

- Faintness, with great flushing of upper part of body and pains in back.

- Swelling of face and legs.

- Burning sensation of lips with free desquamation.

Mouth

- Tongue became thickly coated.

- Feverish and thirsty.

- Great thirst.

- Ulcerated patch on buccal aspect on l. check near angle of mouth.

Throat

- Goitre, exophthalmic, cured.

Respiratory System

- Dormant phthisis ; lighted up the disease in five cases.

Heart and Pulse

- Death, with all symptoms of angina pectoris.

- Frequent fainting fits.

- Sensation of faintness and nausea.

- Palpitation on stooping.

- Rapid pulsation, with inability to lie down in bed.

- Jumping sensation at heart.

Gastro-intestinal System

- Loss of appetite.
- Increased appetite with improved digestion.
- Eructations.
- Dyspeptic troubles.
- Nausea, with flushing and lumbar pains.
- Always felt a sensation of sickness after the injections.
- Sensation of faintness and nausea (after a few injections).
- Gastro-intestinal disturbance and diarrhoea.
- flatulence increased, followed later in the case by amelioration.
- Headache and pain in abdomen.
- Diarrhoea, with gastro-intestinal disturbance.
- Constipation.

Urinary System

- Increase flow of urine.
- Albuminuria.
- Diabetes mellitus ; caused and cured.

Female Reproductive System

- Increased sexual desire.
- Menses profuse, prolonged, more frequent ; early amenorrhoea,
- Painful irregular menstruation.
- Constant left ovarian pain, and great tenderness.
- Acts as a galactagogue when milk is deficient ; when a deficiency is associated with a return of the menses it will suppress the latter.

- Puerperal insanity with fever.
- Puerperal eclampsia.

Back

- Stabbing pains in lumbar region.
- Flushing of upper part of body and pains in back.

Upper Limbs

- Arms less stiff and painful (psoriasis).

Lower Limbs

- Tingling sensation in legs.
- Oedema of legs appeared, and subsequently subsided and continued to reappear and subside for a month.
- Pain in legs.
- Incomplete paraplegia.
- Swelling of face and legs.
- Profuse flow of fluid from feet (in case of dropsy cured by Thyr.)
- Intense aching in back and limbs, lasting three days.
- Pains in arms and legs, with malaise.
- Skin of hands and feet desquamated.
- Acromegaly, subjective symptoms.

Skin

- Flushing of skin.
- Psoriasis : eruption extended and increased.
- Lupus : tight feeling, heat, anrgy redness removed ; suppuration increased.
- Eczema : irritation of skin markedly allayed.
- Teething eczema.
- Syphilitic psoriasis.

- Rupia.
- Scleroderma.
- Peeling of skin of lower limbs, with gradual clearing (eczema).
- Skin of hands and feet desquamated.

Sleep

- Continual tendency to sleep.
- Insomnia.
- Excited condition ; could not sleep.

Fever

- Flushing ; with nausea ; with loss of consciousness.
- Profuse perspiration on least exertion.

Generalities

- malaise > by lying in bed.
- Stooping-Palpitation.
- Rest in recumbent positon > extreme breathlessness with lividity, felt as if dying.
- Myxoedematous patients are always chilly ; the effect of the treatment is to make them less so.
- Loss of consciousness for an hour; next day felt better and warmer.
- Malaise so great she refused to continue the treatment.
- Hysterical attack.
- Hystero-epilepsy with amenorrhoea.
  Aching pains all over.
- Aching pains in various parts of body.
- Lost weight enormously (many cases of myxoedema.
- Anaemia and debility.

- Acromegaly, headache and subjective symptoms.
- Fractures refuse to unite.
- A peculiar cachexia more dangerous than myxoedema itself.
- Syphilis, secondary, tertiary.

USTILAGO

Ustilago Maidis   *Corn-smut*

Mental Generals

- Depression of spirits in afternoon.
- Very sad, cries frequently;exceedingly prostrated from sexual abuse and loss of semen ; sleep restless.
- The day seemed like a dream.
- Melancholia ; depression of spirits ; oppression and faintness in a warm room. An aversion to or < from warmth in general.
- Partial or complete loss of control over the functions of vision and deglutition.
- Great irritability, mental weakness and depression.

Head

- Vertigo at climaxis with too frequent and profuse menstruation.
- Nervous headache from menstrual irregularities in nervous women.
- Bursting congestive sensation to the head ; and various parts of the body.
- Feeling of fulness with dull pressive headache < by walking.

- The headache and vertigo appear to be reflex from ovarian or uterine condition.
- Frontal headache, < by walking.
- Falling of the hair and nails; complete alopecia not a hair on the head.
- Headache in temples.

Eyes

- Spasms, with vanishing of vision and head seems to whirl.
- Aching in eyes and lachrymation.
- Aching and smarting in eyeballs, with profuse secretion of tears.
- Weakness of eyes.
- Dull aching pain in r.eyeball.

Nose

- Bright epistaxis. > pressure.

Face

- Burning of face scalp from congestion.

Teeth

- Sometimes looseness of teeth.
- Aching all day in decayed upper first and second molars, which have ached before.

Mouth

- Salivation ; thin bitter ; profuse.
- Taste : coppery ; in morning : slimy coppery.
- Slimy : slimy with burning distress in stomach.

Chest

- Drawing pain in 1. inframammary region, waking him at 3 A.M., > turning on back from r. side.

Heart

- Burning pain in cardiac region.

Respiratory System

- Feeling as if there were lump behind larynx, which produces constant inclination to swallow.

Appetite

- Appetite : craving ; poor.
- Thirst at night.
- Loss of appetite followed by canine hunger.

Gastro-intestinal System

- Eructations : of sour fluid ; of sour food.
- Cutting in stomach.
- Pain in epigastrium with drawing pain in joints of fingers.
- Haematemesis : passive, venous, accompanied by nausea, which is > by vomiting.
- Weak, empty, all-gone sensation in the stomach.
- Constant distress in region of stomach.
- Burning distress in sternum and stomach, accompanied by fine neuralgic pains in same region, lasting about three minutes at a time ; come on every ten or fifteen minutes for several hours ; sharp cutting pain in stomach.
- Periodical cutting in umbilical and hypogastric regions at 6 P.M., < at 8 P.M. by a constipated stool, afterwards grumbling pain in whole abdomen.
- Pain in r. lobe of liver ; in umbilicus ; in umbilicus before natural stool : in l. groin when walking.
- Grumbling pains in abdomen all afternoon, follwed by dry, hard stool, fine cutting colicky pains every few minutes all day, > by hard constipated stool, followed by dull distress in bowels.

- Light-colored diarrhoea.
- Constipated : black, dry, lumpy stools.

Urinary System

- Tenesmus of bladder and incontinence of urine.

Male Sexual System

- Spermatorrhoea after onanism : emissions every night, talking about woman causes an emission ; very sad ; cries frequently ; say he cannot break off habit, has no control of himself when passion is aroused ; knows it is fast killing him; cannot work, is so prostrated.
- Genitals relaxed.
- Erections : when reading at 4 o'clock ; frequently during day and night.
- Scrotum relaxed and cold sweat on it.
- Pain in testes, < r.
- esire depressed.
- Chronic orchitis, irritable testicle.
- Erotic fancies.
- Seminal emission and irresistible tendecy to masturbation. irresistible tendency to onanism ; frequent emissions ; is prostrated dull, with lumbar backache. Despondent ; irritable.
- Irritable weakness and relaxation of the male sexual organs with erotic fancies and seminal emissions.

Female Reproductive System

- Yellow and offensive leucorrhoea.
- Tenderness of l. ovary, with pain and sweliing.
- Burning distress in ovaries.
- Intermittent neuralgia of l. ovary ; enlarged, very tender to touch.

- Uterus : hypertrophied : prolapsed ; cervix sensitive, spongy.
- Menses : too scanty with ovarian irritation ; too profuse and too early ; blood clotted ; as if everything would come through.
- Between periods constant suffering under l. breast at margin of ribs.
- Oozing of dark blood, highly coagulated, forming occasionally long, black, stringy clots.
- Extreme pain during period ; flow very profuse and did not cease entirely until next period ; most of time confined to bed.
- Suppression of menses.
- Vicarious menstruation from lungs and bowels.
- Constant aching distress at mouth of womb.
- Menorrhagia at climaxis ; active and constant flowing with frequent clots.
- Bland leucorrhoea.
- Abortion.
- Deficient labour pains ; of soft, pliable dilatable.
- Lochia too profuse, partly fluid, partly clotted ; prolonged bearing-down pains ; uterus feels drawn into a knot.
- Hypertrophy and subinvolution of uterus with great atony.
- Metrorrhagia, with vertigo during climacteric.
- Menorrhagia, with displaced uterus.
- Flabby, relaxed condition of pelvic organs, a tonic condition of uterus ; a state of weakness, relaxtion and atony.
- Flushes of heat, and disturbances of circulation similar to

those occurring at the climaxis, or from premature suppression of the menses ; ovaries inflamed, irritable, sensitive and swollen; burning distress in both ovaries.

- Metrorrhagia after miscarriage, confinement or at the climaxis.

- Discharge of blood on the slightest provocation ; after digital or mechanical examination ; cervix swollen, bleeding easily when touched.

- Uterus remains large after miscarriage or confinement ; subinvolution delayed.

- Haemorrahage bright red but more frequently dark, clotted and stringly post-partum oozing from flabby atonic uterus.

- Uterus hypertrophied, heavy, feels soft, spongy or boggy.

- Complaints of the lying-in woman ; profuse debilitating lochia.

- Milk deficient or superabundant ; nursing increases the lochial discharge.

- Acute pain < in l. ovary, with swelling ; pains intermittent; shoot rapidly down legs.

- Ovaritis, constant pains in ovary, sharp pains passing down Legs rapidly ; ovary much swollen and tender, with scanty menstruation.

- Ovaritis ; took cold after menstruation ; constant dull pain in r. groin and back, three or four times an hour; sharp neuralgic pain in ovary : walking painful ; bowels torpid, very languid.

- Ovarian irritation, constant pain in l. ovary passing down hip, has to limp when walking ; pains sharp and at times pass down leg with great rapidity ; every few days has quite a swelling in l. groin ; cannot bear pressure over ovary.

- Displaced uterus with menorrhagia ; cervix tumefied; bleeds when touched.

- Uterus hypertrophied, sensitive, blood bright, fresh, without coagula.

- Subserous or interstitial fibroid of uterus (two cases), fibroid much diminished.

- Cervix tumefied, bleeds when touched.

- For days oozing of dark blood with small coagula ; uterus enlarged, cervix tumefied or dilated.

- Chronic uterine haemorrhage, and passive congestion.

- Blood dark, but so thin as to scarcely colour fingers.

- Profuse menstruation, flow lasting from ten days to two weeks, at first very abundant, gradually wearing off ; always < from motion ; discharge dark and quite pain-less.

- Menses every three weeks, with dark coagulum ; pro-fuse, with gushes of bright-red blood when rising from a seat or after having been startled or frightened; two days before menses, a heavy backache with sharp pain across abdomen from hip to hip, followed by expulsive pains ; pains diminish after flow commence and stop with it ; between menstrual periods heavy dragging backache on exertion : pain shooting up back from hips to shoulder ; abdomen tender to touch ; excessive bearing down ; pressure in head ; sensation of contraction in vertex, and feeling as if head were lifting off ; vertigo ; excoriating albuminous leucorrhoea,<before menses ; ravenous ap-petite; excessive tired feeling ; pulse 80 and weak ; mental depression.

- Subject to profuse menstruation ; childless ; large, fleshy, flabby, bloated-looking, with a very sallow complexion, inclined to be (and formerly had been) dropsical from excessive loss of blood ; profuse menstruation, which seems to her to be principally water and clots ; says there is no outward flow when she lies still, but clots and water pass out of uterus when she gets up ; feels so fully in uterus that she must rise to get rid of clots; flowed fearfully during night ; very low, scarcely able to speak aloud.

- Severe menorrhagia for past twelve years at every menstrual period, lasting a week or ten days, sometimes longer ; pale, thin, weak, very nervous.

- Profuse discharge of dark, clotted blood of foetid odour, with pain and tenderness in one or both ovaries.

- Dysmenorrhoea of a congestive character, with much ovarian irritation ; severe pain in ovaries, uterus and back every few minutes : scanty, pale flow accompanied by false membrances ; poor appetite, thickly-coated tongue.

- Subject to headaches ever since menstruation appeared at age of fifteen ; headache mostly on top of head ; appetite poor ; pain in l. chest with some cough ; total suppression of menses for last eight months ; severe pain in back, is unable to ride in carriage ; pain in uterine region, especially over ovarian region, < l. side ; vomiting of mucus and blood daily ; no sleep ; some leucorrhoea; hysterical ; no uterine displacement, but great congestion in pelvic region.

- Suppression of menses without apparent cause ; troublesome cough ; considerable expectoration ; sometimes also dry cough ; stitching pains in chest, expecially l. side; night sweats ; loss of appetite ; pain in ovaries, especially l.; general debility, headache ; leucorrhoea ; chlorotic ; anaemic, as if in first stage of consumption.

- Menses suppressed for last fourteen months ; very irritable and depressed : uneasiness in region of stomach;

pain in ovarian region ; especially l. : skin hot and dry ; constipation, stools dry and hard ; no appetite : stitching pains in chest, < worse in l. side; constant hacking cough ; considerable expectoration; night sweats ; general prostration ; great uneasiness in lower extremities.

- Climaxis : vertigo ; frequent flushing ; metrorrhagia.

Pregnancy, Parturition, Lactation

- Abortion ; bearing-down pains, as if everything would come from her ; in flabby constitutions ; from general atony of uterus ; with or without haemorrhage.

- Has aborted a number of times at third month; is now about three months pregnant; for last ten days has had more or less haemorrhage every day, some days quite bad ; not so much at night ; blood passes a number of times through day, in dark-colored clots.

- Post-partum haemorrhages from a flabby, atonic condition of uterus.

- Constant flooding ; every few minutes, expulsion of a large clot of bright red blood, with bearing-down pains.

- Persistent haemorrhage of brownish blood, with want of uterine contraction.

- One and a half hours after delivery commenced to flow violently.

- Passive haemorrhage of brownish blood in lumps, flooding for days and weeks.

- Severe flooding two weeks after labour; large bright-red clots; no pain; very weak.

- Very profuse lochial discharge, very dark in colour, almost black.

- Agalactia; chronic inflammation, and induration of mamma.

- Galactorrhea.

- Promotes expulsion of foreign bodies from the uterus.

- Puerperal peritonitis; with constant flooding; high fever; secretion putrid; abdomen excessively tender and tympanitic.

- Puerperal peritonitis; aborted about two days since, at about three months; constant fever; pulse 120; cannot bear least pressure on any portion of bowels; sbout six times today has had sharp, cutting pains in 1. ovary; has flowed constantly for two days; blood dark, not copious, nor attended with bearing-down pains; cannot move in bed; is compelled to lie upon her back; constant, dull, frontal headache; loss of appetite, tongue furred.

- Fibroids and induration of os.

- Discharge of blood from uterus, bright-red, partly fluid, partly clotted; passive congestion of uterus, so that there is a slight oozing of blood after each examination; tissues of uterus feel soft and spongy ; as patulous.

Back

- Pain in back extending to extreme end of spine.

- Severe rheumatic pain in lumbar region, < by walking; aching distress in small of back.

- Pain in back of neck.

- Pain in region of r. kidney, < sitting still; next day in region of l. kidney, > moving about, with heat, fulness, soreness on deep pressure (but it relieved the pain), with uneasiness in l. thigh, frequent desire to urinate, stream very small, the following day it requires considerable effort of will to empty the bladder, which is done slowly, pain and soreness in l. loin continue; heavy in lumbar region, in bed with uneasiness about bladder (had no desire to urinate on going to bed), awake early in morning with distended feeling in bladder, micturition slow and difficult, urine scarcely coloured, pain in back < next night, < lying on face, > lying on r. side.

- Bearing down in sacral region as in dysmenorrhoea, changing to l. ovarian region and gradually extending through hip.

Upper Limbs

- Pain in both shoulders, especially in raising arms.
- Pain in shoulder joint; rheumatic, in muscles of r. shoulder, all night.
- Intermittent, numb tingling sensation in r. arm and hand every day.
- Pain in r. elbow, < by motion.
- Rheumatic drawing pain in finger-joints, < second joint of r. index, all afternoon.
- Hypertrophy or loss of nails.
- Rheumatic pains in arms, hands and fingers.

Lower Limbs

- Pain in l. knee when walking, increasing to cramp, obliging him to lean upon the arm of a friend; the pain, with occasional cramps, lasted all the evening, < raising foot so as to press upon toes.
- Cramp-like stiffness in l. leg, < raising foot so as to press upon toes.
- Rheumatic pains in legs.
- Flying rheumatic pains in metatarsal bones of r. foot.
- Great pains in bones all over body, and especially in calves which are somewhat cramped.

Skin

- Tendency to small boils.

- Boils on nape.
- Skin dry and hot ; congested.
- Painful, destructive disease of nails.
- Paresthesia of the skin; pricking, burning, itching, a marked erythema of skin of the uncovered parts of the body, followed by, a parchment-like, dark brown skin with rhagades < by warmth.
- Copper-colored spots on skin; secondary syphilis; macula.
- Negro, urticaria of six years' standing, troubled more or less all the time; every night itching, scratching parts produce large pale welts on body, arms and legs.

Sleep

- Difficult falling asleep and then unpleasant dreams.
- Sexual dreams; without emission; and disgusting, waking him, arose and urinated with difficulty and tenesmus.

Fever

- Chills running up and down back.
- Heat at night, during sleep.
- Internal heat ; with vertigo; < eyes, which are inflamed and sensitive to light, eyeball sore to touch; intermittent; pulse normal.

Generalities

- Neuralgic pains in forehead, hands and feet.
- Rheumatic pains all up and down l. side, with cutting in l. knee and calf if I pressed any weight upon toes or flexed knee with any weight upon it.

Relations - Compare : Meli., Med., Mez., Psor., Vinc-m., in crusta lactea and other scalp affections of child-hood. Bry., Ham., Mill., Phos., in vicarious menstruation; Agar., Murx.,

Sep., in bearing down and uteine collapse; Helon., Lyss., Sec., delayed subinvolution; Malan., Sec.,affections of the hair and nails; Cimic., Caul., Thuja, Sulph., Vib-o., in l. ovarian pain; Bov., Elaps., Graph., Ham., in intermittent flow; Sang. Urt-u., pain and rheumatic affections of r. shoulder; Sang., l. inframammary pain extending to scapula ; Lac-c., Kali-n., Puls., erratic rheumatic pains; Sulph., faint all gone sensation at 11 A.M.; Cob., backache and seminal emissions; Bou., flow midway between the periods; Canth., Pyrog., Sec., in expelling from the uterus.

VACCININUM

A Nosode from Vaccine matter

Mental Generals

- Crying.
- Ill-humour, with restless sleep.
- Nervous depression, impatient, irritable; disposition to be troubled by things.
- Morbid fear of taking small-pox.
- Confusion, she does not remember things at the time she wants them.

Head

- Frontal headache.
- Forehead felt as if it would split in two in median line from root of nose to top of head.
- Stitches in r. temple.
- Severe headache all over head.
- Prickling in l. temple, as if going to sleep.

Eyes

- Tinea tarsi and conjunctivitis in a woman, age. 28, remaning as result fo variola in infancy, conjunctiva painfully sensitive.
- Weak eyes; falling out in forehead as if it were split.
- Keratitis after vaccination.
- Pain in forehead and eyes as if spilt.
- Glossy sensation before eyes in morning, cannot see well.

Nose

- Full feeling of head, with running of nose.
- Bleeding at nose preceded by feeling of contraction above and between eye-brows, soon after eating meat; menses rather profuse and too frequent ; cured by revaccination.

Neck

- Swelling of the neck under right ear (parotid gland) with sensation like being cut.

Face

- Redness and distension of face, chill running down back, till afternoon.

Mouth

- Dry mouth and tongue.

Respiratory System

- Whooping-cough.

Chest

- stitches in r. side under short ribs in front from r. to l. then a corresponding place l. side, but from l. to r., lasting five minutes, felt in liver and spleen.

Heart

- Aching at heart.

Appetite

- Appetite gone, disgust to taste, smell, and appearance of food.
- Coffee tastes sour.
- Good appetite.

Gastro-intestinal System

- aching in pit of stomach, with short breath.
- A stitch in hepatic region, at margin of last lower rib, axillary line.
- Stitch in splenic region.
- Blown up with flatulence.

Urinary System

- Nephritis with albuminuria, haematuria, and dropsy, developed eleven days after vaccination ; child recovered.

Back

- Backache.
- Aching pain in back, < in lumbar region extending around waist.
- Twisting pain in lower back.
- Weakness in small of back coming on suddenly > by lying down.

Upper Limbs

- Rheumatic pains in wrists and hands.

Lower Limbs

- Soreness of lower extremities, as if heated or over-exerted.
- Twisting pains in both knees.

Skin

- A general eruption similar to cow-pox.

- Small pimples develop at point of vaccination with fourth dilution.

- Red pimples or blotches in various parts, most evident when warm.

- Eruption of pustules with a dark-red base and roundish or oblong elevation, filled with pus of a greenish-yellow colour, at l. side of trunk, between shoulder, on l. shoulder, behind r. ear, resembling varioloid, some as large as a pea, some less without depression in the centre, coming with a round, hard feel in the skin (like a shot), very itchy.

- Vaccininum 200th quickly > severe symptoms of variola occurring in a child, age. six months ; two days before appearance of eruption had been re-vaccinated (after an interval of eight days) on a naevus near r. nipple ; deglutition difficult through implication of tongue and fauces ; pustules, many of large size, scattered over scalp, face, body and limbs.

- Eruption of small, r. vesicles on left upper arm and chest dying off after a few days.

- Pustule filled with matter, with a depression in centre and red halo on l. shoulder.

- Pustules suddenly much depressed.

- Eruption all over body of small pustules, some with a central depression, some brown.

Generalities

- Restlessness.

- General malaise.

- Languor, lassitude.

- Tired all over, with stretching, gaping feeling ; unnatural fatigue.
- Child wants to be carried.
- Many persons faint when being vaccinated.
- Weakness.

PROVINGS OF THE X-RAY

Mental Generals
- Mental irritability.
- Clearing up of mental function after sharp stabbing pain in left temple staggering him, the heart feeling the impulse immediately.
- Mental processes not clear, writes wrong words in letter.
- Mental condition upset during profuse menstruation, would like to kill somebody.

Head
- Sleepy with headache.
- Headache gradually extending to frontal region, worse in centre of forehead.
- Sense of pressure in centre of forehead.
- Dull headache in morning, worse when stooping and after rising.
- Headache and soreness, worse toward afternoon.
- Head feels empty as though scraped, worse at night in bed.
- Pain in right side of head above temple.
- Sharp stabbing in left temple, followed by clearing up mental function, the heart immediately feling the impulse.

- Sense of pressive fulness starting from posterior prominence of vertex in a central straight line to bridge of nose, followed by fulness in entire vertex extending to bridge of nose.

- Aggravation of fulness over vertex, worse along the centre to nose and when stooping over.

- Aching on top of head across a long coronal suture on blowing nose and after it.

- Constant ache in vertex, worse on awaking also on coughing, sneezing, or head low.

- Heavy pressure on vertex as from a hand (old symptom, absent a year).

- Sticking pains in different parts of head and face.

- Cannot bear slightest touch though hard pressure relieves for an instant ; > by walking the floor.

- Pain > by lying on left side of face and body.

- Pain in back of head > at times by massage slightly, also by heat.

- Neuralgic pains.

Neck

- stiffness on left side of neck, turning in bed.

- Stiffness on right side of neck, with intense pain at night; occurs in paroxysms during the day > somewhat by hot applications.

- Sudden "cricks" attack first on side of neck, then the other, < on getting cold turning the head nearly produces convulsions. Pains more severe behind the ears-the mastoid process.

- Pain relieved on keeping perfectly quiet; sometimes by gentle stinging contraction pain.

Eyes
- Eyeballs sore.
- Sensation in right eye as if bulging.

Ears
- fulness in ears, worse in right ear, worse by inserting finger.
- Intermittent noise as of deep steam-whistle in left ear, and ringing in head.
- Ears more clear from ringing and dulness of hearing than for many years, an improvement lasting up to this day. Healing action.

Nose
- Bloody mucus from the nose.
- Sulphur-vapour sensation in throat and nose.
- Congested sensation in head and nose as before coryza.

Face
- Slight electric current sensation in left side of tongue and face passing over and disappearing in right side of face.

Mouth
- Tongue dry, rough, sore and scraped.
- Scrapping pain in lateral incisor, aggravated by noises and jarring of cars.

Throat
- Sulphur-vapour sensation in nose and throat.
- Throat painful on swallowing.

Chest
- Wandering sticking pains in chest, worse on right side.
- Stitching pain in right upper chest going through to upper part of scapula.

Heart

- Palpitation during evening causing cough.
- sharp pain at apex of heart, better by lying on left side.
- Palpitation with a cough with tearing sensation in bronchi and hoarseness.
- Heart's sound keeps him awake while lying on left side.
- Dull and constant soreness around heart, and worse in legs and arms.

Appetite

- Aversion to meat.
- Appetite diminished.
- Desire for sweets.
- Most distress after midday and evening meal.
- No hunger, goes till he feels faint.
- Can eat plenty but does not enjoy it.
- More thirst than usual.
- Thirst for cold drinks though nothing tastes good.
- Bad taste in forenoon.
- Bitter taste.

Gastro-intestinal System

- Nausea and vomiting with profuse sweat after immense stool at 4 A.M. seven days after taking.
- abdomen distended with full feeling. (Pulsatilla, which a year ago helped for months a train of symptoms, had only very slight effect.)
- Flatulence with ineffectual desire for stool.
- Colicky pains in right lower abdomen, sometimes extending behind the hip, and retained urine.

- Stools green, though normal in consistency.
- On straining at stool a sore sensation in nates.
- Ineffectual urine of stool, with flatulence .

Urinary System

- Retained uringe, vesical tenesmus after enormous evacuation, vomiting for twelve hours to 4 P.M.
- Frequent urination, worse after getting into bed.
- Pressure as from congestion about kidneys.

Male Sexual System

- sexual desire lost in man.
- Testes relaxed, impotent feeling.
- Unnatural or disgusting, lewd dream on several nights, or several times in one night.

Female Reproductive System

- Menses dark green one day.
- Pain darting upward in region of left ovary when sitting walking or standing.
- Flushes of heat ; better afternoons and evenings.

Back

- Pain in dorsal region.
- Lame and stiff in back.
- Aching whole length of spine.
- A paralytic sensation extending from spine down left leg.
- Rheumatic-like fever in trunk, steady dull pain going steadily from trunk to legs, and finally to heels, worse in left knee, worse stepping on heel, on underside of heel (old symptom of inflammatory rheumatism twenty-five years ago).

Upper Extremities

- Rheumatic pain in left wrist and forearm.
- Rheumatic twinge in last two phalangeal articulations of index and middle fingers for a short time in fore-noon
- Rheumatic pain in right wrist and arm.
- Can't hold thigns in left hand, powerless or clumsy.
- Palms of hands. which where rough and scaly and bleeding at times, became smooth and natural during the proving. Healing action. (Afterward they went back to former state when general health improved.)

Lower Extremities

- Lower part of both legs asleep, tingling as if from electric battery more in right, immediately.
- Sciatic pain in right hip.
- Rheumatic pains in limbs.
- Dull aching posterior aspect of thigh and calf in morning, from above downward.
- Pain in right sciatic nerve on walking.
- Rheumatic pains in front of right thigh.
- Drawing aching discomfort in right thigh through hip and knees down through toes, immediately.
- Feeling as if somebody were drawing icy hands over thigh downward, aggravatingly slow. (This occurred first twelve years ago after a nervous shock and did not return for five years.)
- Rheumatic like fever in trunk, steady dull pain going steadily down to legs and finally to heels, worse in left knee, worse stepping on heel, on underside of heel (old symptoms of inflammatory rheumatism twenty-five years ago).

Fever

- Chills as soon as beginning to sleep, running up back, preventing sleep.
- Chill going down back, followed by paralytic feeling in right cheek.
- Wave-like sensation as if it would break out in perspiration.
- Profuse perspiration on getting into bed, keeping him awake.

Sleep

- Kept awake by heart's sound while laying on left side.
- As soon as she begins to sleep, chills running up back preventing sleep.
- Sleeplessness constant and troublesome (relieved permanently by a bottle of Pabst Malt Extract).
- Drowsy all night while sitting up.
- Drowsiness leaves the instant when laying down, so cannot sleep.
- Symptoms worse when getting into bed, worse after sunset.
- Profuse perspiration on getting into bed, keeping him awake.
- Sleepy during day.
- Walking frequently at night from no aparent cause.
- all symptoms worse in bed.
- Dreams of strife, busy dreams.
- Very vivid lewd dreams, repeated night after night.

General Symptoms

- General tired and sick feeling.

- Persistent exhaustion and languor, not attributable to spring.
- Lame and sore all over.
- Trembling all over.

Skin

- Reappearance of an old, slight, pimply eruption on left side of forehead.
- Return of a slight eruption on outside of lower legs, burning when scratched, worse after scratching.

Aggravation - In bed; towards evening and at night (both mental and physical); in the open air; in the afternoon.

Relations - Compare : the Calcareas, Caust., Hep, Med., Nat-m., Psor., Puls., Sil., Sulph., Thuja, Tub., for its power to reproduce old or suppressed symptoms and conditions ; Cimic., Lil-t., Lac-c., Plat., Sep., Pyrog., for nervous reflexes and neuralgic conditions from ovearian or uterine irritation : Agar., Cur., Tarent., Zinc., for irritation of th cord, spinal reflexes, neurasthenia; electric storms, thunderstorms, Agar., Med., Nat-c., Phos., Psor., Rhod., Sep., Sil., Syph., Thuja.

Antidotes - Nux-v., Sulph. and the dynamic potencies of the remedy.

Alumina.15, 16, 25,15, 16 ,30, 41, 44, 52, 57, 72, 83, 85, 95, 110, 125, 131, 138, 146, 150, 151, 180, 184, 205, 221, 229, 262, 283, 302, 305.

Ambra grisea. 27, 21, 248, 293.

Ammonium carbonicum. 28, 13, 47, 49, 63, 65, 87, 139, 153, 159, 162, 170, 200, 210, 250, 265, 302.

Ammonium muriaticum. 30, 25, 42, 90, 174, 175, 201.

Amylenum nitrosum. 30, 13, 44, 58, 71, 125, 130, 184, 230.

Anacardium orientale. 32, 26, 52, 53, 78, 79, 101, 125, 136, 152, 161, 164, 166, 207, 215, 229, 232, 272, 297.

KEYNOTES

REARRANGED AND CLASSIFIED

with

LEADING REMDIES OF THE

MATERIA MEDICA

&

BOWEL NOSODES

By

H.C. ALLEN, M.D.

KEYNOTES
REARRANGED AND CLASSIFIED

ABOUT..............
ALLEN'S KEYNOTES
Rearranged and Classified

"Allen's keynotes" is one of the most popular and widely read materia medicas. The reason for its popularity being, its preciseness and comprehensiveness.

Keeping in view, its usefulness for the students and practitioners of homoeopathy, the ninth edition has been brought out with certain changes.

In the previous editions, the symptoms do not conform to any order and are randomly placed. They also do not follow each other in a logical sequence.

In this edition, all the symptoms belonging to one organ or organs having a similiar and related function, are grouped together, so as to facilitate a deeper understanding of the pathogenesis of a drug and the genesis of a symptom.

For eg:- faecal vomiting is normally listed under the heading-**Stomach**. But the primary cause of faecal vomiting is, intestinal obstruction. Hence instead of using the conventional headings **Stomach, Abdomen, Rectum, Stool,** used frequently in various materia medicas, the heading Gastro-intestinal system has been used. This is because all the organs of the **GIT** are related, as they serve a common function, albiet in different stages.

Also some of the abbreviations used in the previous editions were outdated and pointed to more than one remedies. All the abbreviations used in this edition are standardized according to the SYNTHESIS.

The symptoms are unaltered in substance and the language remains unchanged. The difference between this edition and the previous editions is that the symptoms have been re-arranged and now follow each other in a logical sequence, so that no symptom is lost to the reader even on casual reading.

The fact remains that Dr. Allen had left an indestructible monument of the homoeopathic materia medica, one that is true to its science and immensely useful to anyone who consults it.

B. JAIN PUBLISHERS (PVT.) LTD.

1921, Chuna Mandi, Street No. 10th
Post Box 5775, Paharganj
New Delhi - 110 055
Ph.: 7536418, 3670430, 3670572
Fax: 91-11-3610471, 7536420
Email: bjain@vsnl.com.
Website: www.bjainindia.com